The New Blue Zone Diet

The Definitive Diet

Shirlene V. Moore

Contents

1. Introduction — 1

2. The Blue Zones are five regions — 3

3. What Are Blue Zones, and What Are Their Benefits? — 5

4. What Is the Blue Zone Diet, and Why Should You Try It? — 7

5. Where do the Blue Zones exist? — 9

6. The Blue Zone Diet includes a variety of foods. — 11

7. Greens with a lot of colour — 13

8. Extra Virgin Olive Oil is a type of extra virgin — 15

9. Steel-Cut Oatmeal — 17

10. Blueberries — 19

11. Barley — 21

12. Dietary Guidelines for the Blue Zones — 23

13. How you can do it — 25

14.

Protein in the Blue Zones Diet: A Few Points to Consider   27

15. Consume up to three ounces of fish every day   33

16. Eggs on Occasion   37

17. Daily Dose of Beans   39

18. Bread with a tangy flavor   47

19. Daily Dose of Beans   53

20. Bread with a tangy flavor   61

21. Four Always   75

22. Nuts besides almonds   81

23. It's time to celebrate.   85

24. Pasta with Cherry Tomatoes and Basil in One Pot in the Instant Pot   89

25. Salad of Sardinian oranges and fennel with citrus vinaigrette   91

26. NICOYA CHUNKY VEGAN SOUP   95

27. Conclusion   97

Chapter One

Introduction

Obesity and disease rates are rising, as are eating habits. So, what if the solution is to completely abandon "slimming down"? The majority of popular diets fall short of expectations. This is due to a lack of certain food varieties or even entire food groups, making it difficult to maintain a long-term diet. The ketogenic diet, for example, is the subject of intense debate because, while many people report immediate success, research suggests that there are more practical and viable long-term options. Most diets are similar in that they focus on a quick fix rather than behavior change and evaluating food relationships. Rather than eating (or restricting) to lose weight, we should eat food varieties that promote longevity... because, as it turns out, this way of eating also promotes weight gain. It is my job as an enlisted dietitian to sort through the evidence in order to provide accurate and up-to-date nutrition advice, but this can quickly become overwhelming due to the constant

2 THE NEW BLUE ZONE DIET

flux of information in nutrition's "youthful" science. I was recently given a cookbook called The Blue Zones Kitchen, which is structured similarly to evidence-based nutrition but with excellent photographs, stories, and tried-and-true recipes.

Chapter Two

The Blue Zones are five regions

The Blue Zones are five regions around the world where people live the longest:

Sardinia is an Italian island that is located off the coast of the Mediterranean Sea. Japan's Okinawa Costa Rica's Nicoya is one of the most beautiful places in the world. Greece (Ikaria)

California's Loma Linda is a suburb of Los Angeles.

What better way to learn about the best diet than to look at the diets of people who live to be 100? While the diets are similar in these regions, so are the lifestyles – little to no technology or mechanical conveniences, frequent movement, time spent with family and friends, and, most importantly, a sense of purpose. It's known as ikigai in Okinawa and plan de vida in Nicoya. "A sense of responsibility: for their community, family, or the next generation" is present in the lives of blue zone residents. These ideas emphasize the importance of mental health, a sense of belonging, and getting together as a community to cook, eat, and enjoy life. It's a straightforward way of life that extends to their eating habits. Dietary restrictions, calorie counting, or the use of meal replacement shakes are not practiced by Blue Zone residents. They eat fresh produce from their gardens, occasionally eat meat and fish, and drink red wine with their meals.

Chapter Three

What Are Blue Zones, and What Are Their Benefits?

Dan Buettner, a National Geographic Fellow and author, set out in the early 2000s on a quest to learn the secrets to living a long life. He discovered five distinct places in the world where people live the longest, healthiest lives at the end of a decade-long research period: Ikaria, Greece; Loma Linda, California; Sardinia, Italy; Okinawa, Japan; and Nicoya, Costa Rica. These areas have been dubbed "blue zones" by Buettner, who has written a book called "The Blue Zones Solution" about them. Despite the fact that climate plays a role, Buettner discovered that these super-agers all have one thing in common: a healthy diet. A plant-based diet is one in which meat is consumed no more than five times per month. According to CNN, Buettner and his team have begun deploying Blue Zones Project communities, with Albert Lea, Minnesota, as the first. Albert Lea residents gained 2.9 years of life extension and saved millions of dollars in healthcare costs as a result of the Blue Zones Project's lifestyle changes. Dan Buettner, a National Geographic Fellow and author, set out in the early 2000s on a quest to discover the secrets of aging. He discovered five distinct places in the world where people live the longest, healthiest lives at the end of a decade-long research period: Ikaria, Greece; Loma Linda, California; Sardinia, Italy; Okinawa, Japan; and Nicoya, Costa Rica. These areas have been dubbed "blue zones" by Buettner, who has written a book called "The Blue Zones Solution" about them. Despite the fact that climate plays a role, Buettner discovered that these super-agers all have one thing in common: they eat well. A plant-based diet is one in which meat is consumed no more than five times per month. According to CNN, Buettner and his team have begun deploying Blue Zones Project communities, with Albert Lea, Minnesota, as the first. Albert Lea residents gained 2.9 years of life extension and saved millions of dollars in healthcare costs as a result of the Blue Zones Project's lifestyle changes.

Chapter Four

What Is the Blue Zone Diet, and Why Should You Try It?

It will help you lose weight and live longer, but it is not a fad diet.

The anti-inflammatory benefits of Blue Zone individuals' dietary choices, according to research, are a powerful mechanism behind their longevity and reduction of ongoing sickness. While these centenarians aren't all vegans, plants are a big part of their weight-loss plans. Blue Zone residents place a high value on vegetables, particularly those grown at home, as they provide a wealth of vitamins, minerals, fiber, and antioxidants. In these populations, beans and lentils are excellent plant-based protein sources. Vegetables, like fruits, contain a high amount of fiber, which has a variety of health benefits, including lowering the risk of cardiovascular disease and aiding in blood sugar control. Solid fats like olive oil, which are high in heart-healthy fatty acids and antioxidants, are used in a few Blue Zone regions. People in the blue zone eat less red meat and only three times per week eat small portions of fish. These people still eat sweets and other types of food in moderation, but they eat sensibly and don't overindulge. Weight is kept under control and obesity is not as prevalent to fuel persistent disease by maintaining balance and equilibrium with food choices, especially by adhering to rules like the hara hachi bu principle used by the Okinawans.

Chapter Five

Where do the Blue Zones exist?

Sardinia, Italy: Sardinia is the Mediterranean Sea's second-largest island, and it is home to some of the world's oldest men. Local shepherds walk at least five mountainous miles every day and eat mostly plants. Sundays and special occasions are the only times when meat is consumed.

Okinawa, Japan: Okinawa, a chain of Japanese islands, is home to the world's oldest women. Their long lives are attributed in part to their close social circles, as well as an old Confucian mantra recited before meals to remind them not to overeat and to stop when they are 80 percent full.

Residents of Loma Linda, California, have one of the highest rates of longevity in the United States. The Seventh-Day Adventist community in Loma Linda eats mostly vegan food and observes the Sabbath on a weekly basis.

Nicoya, Costa Rica: The Nicoya Peninsula is known for its positive elders. Their diet is high in antioxidant-rich tropical fruits, and their water is high in calcium and magnesium, which aids in the prevention of heart disease and the development of strong bones.

Ikaria, Greece is known for its long-lived residents who eat a Mediterranean diet rich in olive oil, fruits, vegetables, whole grains, and beans. A mid-afternoon break is also taken by Ikarians. Heart disease is half as common in them as it is in Americans, and they have 20% fewer cancer cases. Furthermore, the majority of Ikarians are Greek Orthodox Christians who fast several times a year and eat a vegan diet.

Chapter Six

The Blue Zone Diet includes a variety of foods.

Legumes

Legumes, such as chickpeas and lentils, are an important part of every Blue Zone diet. Legumes are a good source of protein, complex carbohydrates, and a variety of vitamins and minerals. They're also high in fiber and known for their heart-healthy effects. Whether you prefer pinto beans or black-eyed peas, eat a half-cup of legumes every day. Legumes are a versatile ingredient that can be used in salads, soups, stews, and a variety of vegetable-based dishes.

Chapter Seven

Greens with a lot of colour

Dark leafy greens such as kale, spinach, and Swiss chard are particularly prized in the Blue Zone diet. Dark leafy greens, one of the most nutrient-dense vegetables, contain several vitamins, including vitamin A and vitamin C, that have powerful antioxidant properties.

Nuts

Nuts are high in protein, vitamins, and minerals, similar to legumes. They also contain heart-healthy unsaturated fats, and some research suggests that eating nuts can help lower cholesterol levels. According to Feller, "nuts are a high-fiber food." "A one-ounce serving of almonds, for example, contains approximately 3.5 grams of fiber." Try a handful of almonds, walnuts, pistachios, cashews, or Brazil nuts, as Blue Zone residents do, for a healthier snack.

Chapter Eight

Extra Virgin Olive Oil is a type of extra virgin

Olive oil, a staple in Blue Zone diets, is high in health-promoting fatty acids, antioxidants, and compounds like oleuropein. Olive oil has been shown in numerous studies to benefit heart health in a variety of ways, including lowering cholesterol and blood pressure. Furthermore, new research suggests that olive oil may aid in the prevention of diseases such as Alzheimer's and diabetes. Select the extra-virgin variety of olive oil as often as possible, and use your oil for cooking and in salads and vegetable dishes. Olive oil is sensitive to light and heat, so be sure to store it in a cool, dark area like a kitchen cabinet.

Chapter Nine

Steel-Cut Oatmeal

When it comes to whole grains, those in Blue Zones often choose oats. One of the least processed forms of oats, steel-cut oats make for a high-fiber and incredibly filling breakfast option. Although they're perhaps best known for their cholesterol-lowering power, oats may also provide plenty of other health benefits. For instance, recent research has determined that oats may thwart weight gain, fight diabetes, and prevent hardening of the arteries.

Chapter Ten

Blueberries

Fresh fruit is the go-to sweet treat for many people living in Blue Zones. While most any type of fruit can make for a healthy dessert or snack, foods such as blueberries may offer bonus benefits. For example, recent studies have demonstrated that blueberries may help shield your brain health as you age. But the benefits might go even further. Other research says blueberries might fend off heart disease by improving blood pressure control.

Chapter Eleven

Barley

Another whole grain favored in Blue Zones, barley may possess cholesterol-lowering properties similar to those of oats, according to a study published in the European Journal of Clinical Nutrition. Barley also delivers essential amino acids, as well as compounds that may help stimulate digestion.

Chapter Twelve

Dietary Guidelines for the Blue Zones

Follow these guidelines and you'll crowd out refined starches and sugar, replace them with more wholesome, nutrient-dense, and fiber-rich foods—and do it all naturally.

Slant of the Plant

See that 95 percent of your food comes from a plant or a plant product. Limit animal protein in your diet to no more than one small serving per day. Favor beans, greens, yams and sweet potatoes, fruits, nuts, and seeds. Whole grains are okay too. While people in four of the five Blue Zones consume meat, they do so sparingly, using it as a celebratory food, a small side, or a way to flavor dishes. As our adviser Walter Willett of the Harvard School of Public Health puts it: "Meat is like radiation: We don't know the safe level." Indeed, research suggests that 30-year-old vegetarian Adventists will likely outlive their meat-eating counterparts by as many as eight years. At the same time, increasing the amount of plant-based foods in your meals has many salutary effects. In the Blue Zones people eat an impressive variety of garden vegetables when they are in season, and then they pickle or dry the surplus to enjoy during the off-season. The best of the best longevity foods in the Blue Zones diet are leafy greens such as spinach, kale, beet and turnip tops, chard, and collards. In Ikaria more than 75 varieties of edible greens grow like weeds; many contain ten times the polyphenols found in red wine. Studies have found that middle-aged people who consumed the e q uivalent of a cup of cooked greens daily were half as likely to die in the next four years as those who ate no greens. Researchers have also found that people who consumed a quarter pound of fruit daily (about an apple) were 60 percent less likely to die during the next four years than those who didn't. Many oils derive from plants, and they are all preferable to animal-based fats. We cannot say that olive oil is the only healthy plant-based oil, but it is the one most often used in the Blue Zones diet. Evidence shows that olive oil consumption increases good cholesterol and lowers bad cholesterol. In Ikaria we found that for middle-aged people about six tablespoons of olive oil daily seemed to cut the risk of dying in half. Combined with seasonal fruits and vegetables, whole grains and beans dominate Blue Zones diets and meals all year long.

Chapter Thirteen

How you can do it

Always have a supply of your favorite fruits and veggies on hand. Don't push yourself to consume foods you don't care for. That may work for a time, but it will eventually run out of steam. Try a variety of fruits and veggies; after you've decided the ones you prefer, have them on hand in your kitchen. Frozen vegetables can suffice if you don't have access to fresh, inexpensive vegetables. (In fact, since they're flash-frozen just after harvest rather than traveling for weeks to your local grocer's shelves, they frequently contain more nutrients.)

Use olive oil in the same way you would butter. In a small saucepan, sauté the veggies in olive oil over low heat. Steamed or boiled veggies may also be finished with a drizzle of extra-virgin olive oil, which you should have on hand.

Make sure you have enough of whole grains on hand. Oats, barley, brown rice, and ground maize were seen in Blue Zones diets all around the globe. Wheat did not play as important a part in ancient societies, and the grains they ate had less gluten than current strains.

To create vegetable soup, cut whatever veggies are sitting unused in your fridge, brown them in olive oil and seasonings, and cover with boiling water. Simmer until the veggies are tender, then season with salt and pepper to taste. Freeze anything you don't eat right away in single or family-size containers, then reheat when you don't have time to prepare later in the week or month.

Chapter Fourteen

Protein in the Blue Zones Diet: A Few Points to Consider

We've all been told that protein is necessary for healthy bones and muscular growth, but how much is enough? The typical American woman eats 70 grams of protein per day, whereas the average American guy consumes over 100 grams: this is excessive. The Centers for Disease Control and Prevention suggests consuming 46 to 56 grams of protein each day. However, quantity isn't everything. We also need the proper protein. Protein, commonly known as amino acids, is available in 21 different forms. The body cannot synthesize nine of them, which are referred to as "essential" amino acids since we need them and must get them from our food. All nine amino acids are found in meat and eggs, but only a few plant foods offer them. However, meat and eggs contain fat and cholesterol, which are linked to heart disease and cancer. So, if you want to follow the Blue Zones diet and consume mostly plant-based meals, how do you go about doing it? The key is to "paint" different cuisines together. You can receive all of the needed amino acids by mixing the correct plant sources. You'll satisfy your protein requirements while still limiting your calorie consumption.

Meat should be avoided.

Meat should be consumed no more than twice a week.

Eat meat only once or twice a week, in portions of no more than two ounces cooked. Instead of industrially grown meats, choose authentic free-range chicken and family-farmed hog or lamb. Processed meats such as hot dogs, luncheon meats, and sausages should be avoided.

People in the Blue Zones ate tiny quantities of pork, chicken, or lamb in their diets. (With the exception of Adventists, who ate no meat at all.) For festival festivities, families customarily killed their pig or goat, ate heartily, and kept the leftovers, which they would subsequently use sparingly as fat for frying or as a flavoring spice. Chickens freely wandered the area, grazing on grubs and roosting. Chicken flesh, on the other hand, was a rare luxury that was relished over several meals.

We found that people ate small amounts of meat, about two ounces or less at a time, about five times per month when we averaged meat consumption across all Blue Zones. They splurged around once a month, typically on roasted pig or goat. In the usual Blue Zones diet, neither beef nor turkey play a large role.

Meats from a Free-Range Environment

The meat consumed in the Blue Zones originates from wild animals. These animals are not given hormones, pesticides, or antibiotics, and they are not subjected to the hardships of large feedlots. Goats graze on grasses, leaves, and herbs all day. Pigs from Sardinia and Ikaria consume kitchen leftovers and scavenge for acorns and roots in the wild. Traditional husbandry practices are likely to produce meat with higher levels of beneficial omega-3 fatty acids than grain-fed animals' meat.

Furthermore, we don't know whether people lived longer as a result of eating a small amount of meat as part of the Blue Zones diet or if they thrived in spite of it. Because the Blue Zones individuals participated in so many healthful activities, they may have been able to get away with a little meat now and again because its negative effects were offset by other diet and lifestyle choices. "The more healthy habits you engage in, the healthier you become," says my buddy Dean Ornish.

How to go about it:

Find out what two ounces of cooked beef looks like: Half a chicken breast fillet or the flesh (without the skin) of a chicken leg; Before cooking, cut or slice pork or lamb into the size of a deck of cards.

Beef, hot dogs, luncheon meats, sausages, and other processed meats should not be brought into the home since they are not part of the Blue Zones diet.

Find plant-based alternatives to the meat that is traditionally served in the center of a meal in the United States. Tofu delicately sautéed in olive oil; tempeh, another soy product; or black bean or chickpea cakes are also good options.

Choose two days a week to consume meat or other animal-derived foods, and only eat it on those days.

Because restaurant meat portions are almost always four ounces or more, split meat entrées with a friend or request a container ahead of time so you can take half the meat portion home to eat later.

Protein Combinations You'll Love

Peter J. Woolf, a chemical engineer and former assistant professor at the University of Michigan, collaborated with colleagues to examine over 100 plant-based meals to determine the best pairings and ratios for meeting human protein requirements. Here are some of our favorite meal combinations from the Blue Zones diet.

Snacks That Aren't Too Time Consuming

1 1/2 cups edamame, boiled and seasoned with soy sauce 1 1/2 cups boiled edamame + 1/4 cup walnuts

Blue Zones Diet Low-Calorie Pairings

2 cups chopped carrots + 1 cup cooked lentils 1 1/3 cup chopped red peppers plus 3 cups cooked cauliflower

1 cup cooked chickpeas + 3 cups cooked mustard greens 1 cup lima beans + 2 cups cooked carrots

1 1/4 cup cooked delicious yellow corn + 1 cup cooked black-eyed peas

Blue Zones Diet Dishes that are Extra-Filling

1 1/4 cup brown rice, plus 1 cup chickpeas, cooked

1 1/2 cups broccoli rabe, cooked extra 1 1/3 cup wild rice, cooked 1 cup cooked brown rice + 2/3 cup very firm tofu

1 1/4 cup cooked soba noodles + 1/2 cup firm tofu

It's All Right With Fish

Chapter Fifteen

Consume up to three ounces of fish every day

Before it's cooked, three ounces is about the size of a deck of cards. Choose fish that are plentiful and not endangered by overfishing. The Adventist Health Study 2, which has been tracking 96,000 Americans since 2002, discovered that neither vegans nor meat eaters lived the longest. They were "pesco-vegetarians," or pescatarians, who ate a plant-based diet with a small amount of fish once or twice a day. Fish was a frequent element of regular meals in other Blue Zones diets, with fish being eaten two to three times per week on average. Incorporating fish into your diet comes with additional ethical and health implications. Small, relatively affordable fish like sardines, anchovies, and cod are often consumed throughout the world's Blue Zones—middle-of-the-food-chain species that are not subjected to the high levels of mercury or other pollutants like PCBs that damage our gourmet fish supply today.

People in the Blue Zones do not overfish the waterways in the same way that corporate fisheries do, endangering whole species. Fishermen in the Blue Zones cannot afford to damage the ecosystems on which they rely. However, there is no proof in the Blue Zones diet that any specific fish, including salmon, is beneficial.

How to do it: Learn to recognize three ounces, whether it's three ounces of a larger fish like snapper or trout or three ounces of a smaller fish like sardines or anchovies.

Trout, snapper, grouper, sardines, and anchovies are all good mid-chain species. Avoid predatory fish like swordfish, shark, or tuna if you want to eat like the Blue Zones. Overfished species, such as Chilean sea bass, should be avoided.

Avoid "farmed" fish because they are usually raised in overcrowded pens, necessitating the use of antibiotics, pesticides, and coloring.

Dairy consumption should be reduced.

Consume as little cow's milk and dairy products as possible, such as cheese, cream, and butter. Except for the Adventists, who eat eggs and dairy products, cow's milk does not play a significant role in any Blue Zones diet. Dairy is a very recent addition to the human diet, having been introduced between 8,000 and 10,000 years ago. Our digestive systems are not designed for milk or milk products (other than human milk), and we now know that up to 60% of the population has some difficulty digesting lactose (often unknowingly). The high fat and sugar content of milk is often used as an argument against it. The Physicians Committee for Responsible Medicine's founder and president, Neal Barnard, points out that fat accounts for 49 percent of the calories in whole milk and about 70 percent of the calories in cheese—and that much of this fat is saturated. Lactose sugar is present in every milk. Lactose sugar, for example, accounts for about 55 percent of the calories in skim milk.

While Americans have relied on milk for calcium and protein for decades, the Blue Zones diet relies on plant-based sources for these nutrients. For example, one cup of cooked kale or two-thirds of a cup of tofu has the same amount of bioavailable calcium as a cup of milk. A Blue Zones diet allows for small quantities of sheep's milk or goat's milk products, notably full-fat, naturally fermented yogurt with no added sugars, a few times each week. Both the Ikarian and Sardinian Blue Zones' traditional menus feature goat's and sheep's milk products prominently. We don't know whether it's the goat's milk or sheep's milk that makes humans healthier, or if it's the fact that people in the Blue Zones traverse the same mountainous terrain as goats. Surprisingly, the majority of goat's milk consumed in the Blue Zones diet is fermented products such as yogurt, sour milk, or cheese. Lactose is present in goat's milk, but it also contains lactase, an enzyme that aids in the digestion of lactose.

How to go about it:

As a dairy substitute, try unsweetened soy, coconut, or almond milk. Most have the same amount of protein as regular milk and, in many cases, taste just as good or better.

Cheese made from grass-fed goats or sheep will satisfy your occasional cheese cravings. Try pecorino sardo from Sardinia or feta from Greece. Because they are both rich, only a small amount is required to flavor food.

Chapter Sixteen

Eggs on Occasion

No more than three eggs each week are recommended.

All five Blue Zones diets include eggs, which are ingested two to four times per week on average. The egg, like meat protein, is served as a side dish with a larger portion of whole grain or other plant-based feature. Nicoyans fry an egg before folding it into a corn tortilla with beans on the side. In Okinawan soup, an egg is boiled. For breakfast, people in the Mediterranean Blue Zones fried an egg with bread, almonds, and olives as a side dish. Eggs in the Blue Zones diet originate from hens who are allowed to roam freely, consume a broad variety of natural foods, are not given hormones or antibiotics, and produce eggs that are naturally enriched in omega-3 fatty acids due to their gradual maturation. Factory-produced eggs mature about twice as quickly as eggs laid by Blue Zone breeds of chickens. Eggs are a complete protein source, including all of the essential amino acids as well as B vitamins, vitamins A, D, and E, and minerals like selenium. According to the Adventist Health Study 2, vegetarians who ate eggs lived somewhat longer than vegans (though they tended to weigh more). Other health considerations may impact your choice to include eggs in your Blue Zones diet. Egg intake has been linked to greater risks of prostate cancer in men and aggravated renal issues in women, therefore diabetics should be careful when eating egg yolks. Despite the fact that academics disagree regarding the impact of dietary cholesterol on arteries, some individuals with heart or circulatory issues avoid it.

How to go about it:

Only buy tiny eggs from pastured, cage-free birds.

Fruit or other plant-based items like whole-grain porridge or toast may help round out a one-egg breakfast.

Try substituting scrambled tofu for eggs as part of your Blue Zones diet.

In baking, use a q uarter cup of applesauce, a q uarter cup of mashed potatoes, or a small banana to substitute for one egg. There are also ways to use flaxseeds or agar (extracted from algae) in recipes that call for eggs.

Chapter Seventeen

Daily Dose of Beans

Eat at least a half cup of cooked beans daily.

Beans are the cornerstone of every Blue Zones diet in the world: black beans in Nicoya; lentils, garbanzo, and white beans in the Mediterranean; and soybeans in Okinawa. The long-lived populations in these Blue Zones eat at least four times as many beans as we do, on average. One five-country study, financed by the World Health Organization, found that eating 20 grams of beans daily reduced a person's risk of dying in any given year by about 8 percent . The fact is, beans represent the consummate superfood in the Blue Zones diet. On average, they are made up of 21 percent protein, 77 percent complex carbohydrates (the kind that deliver a slow and steady energy, rather than the spike you get from refined carbohydrates like white flour), and only a few percent fat. They are also an excellent source of fiber. They're cheap and versatile, come in a variety of textures, and are packed with more nutrients per gram than any other food on Earth. Humans have eaten beans for at least 8,000 years; they're part of our culinary DNA. Even the Bible's book of Daniel (1:1-21) offers a two-week bean diet to make children healthier. The Blue Zones dietary average—at least a half cup per day—provides most of the vitamins and minerals you need. And because beans are so hearty and satisfying, they'll likely push less healthy foods out of your diet. Moreover, the high fiber content in beans helps healthy probiotics flourish in the gut.

How you can do it:\sFind ways to cook beans that taste good to you and your family as part of a Blue Zones diet. Centenarians in the Blue Zones know how to make beans taste good. If you don't have favorite recipes already, resolve to try three bean recipes over the next month.

Make sure your kitchen pantry has a variety of beans to prepare. Dry beans are cheapest, but canned beans are q uicker. When buying canned beans, be sure to read the label: The only ingredients should be beans, water, spices, and perhaps a small amount of salt. Avoid the brands with added fat or sugar.

Use pureed beans as a thickener to make soups creamy and protein-rich on the Blue Zones diet.

Make salads heartier by sprinkling cooked beans onto them. Serve hummus or black bean cakes alongside salads for added texture and appeal.

Keep your pantry stocked with condiments that dress up bean dishes and make them taste delicious. Mediterranean bean recipes, for example, usually include carrots, celery, and onion, seasoned with garlic, thyme, pepper, and bay leaves. This is an easy way to mix up a Blue Zones diet.

When you go out to dinner, consider Mexican restaurants, which almost always serve pinto or black beans. Enhance the beans by adding rice, onions, peppers, guacamole, and hot sauce.

Avoid white flour tortillas. Instead, opt for corn tortillas, with which beans are consumed in Costa Rica.

Slash Sugar

Consume no more than seven added teaspoons a day.

Centenarians typically eat sweets only during celebrations. Their foods have no added sugar, and they typically sweeten their tea with honey. This adds up to about seven teaspoons of sugar a day within the Blue Zones diets. The lesson to us: Enjoy cookies, candy, and bakery items only a few times a week and ideally as part of a meal. Avoid foods with added sugar. Skip any product where sugar is among the first five ingredients listed. Limit sugar added to coffee, tea, or other foods to no more than four teaspoons per day. Break the habit of snacking on sugar-heavy sweets. Let's face it: You can't avoid sugar. It occurs naturally in fruits, vegetables, and even milk. But that's not the problem. Between 1970 and 2000, the amount of added sugars in the food supply rose 25 percent . This adds up to about 22 teaspoons of added sugar that the average American consumes daily—insidious, hidden sugars mixed into sodas, yogurts, muffins, and sauces. Too much sugar in our diet has been shown to suppress the immune system, making it harder to fend off diseases. It also spikes insulin levels, which can lead to diabetes and lower fertility, make you fat, and even shorten your life. In the Blue Zones diet, people consume about the same amount of naturally occurring sugars as North Americans do, but only about a fifth as much added sugar. The key: People in the Blue Zones consume sugar intentionally, not by habit or accident.

How you can do it:\sMake honey your go-to sweetener for a Blue Zones diet. Granted, honey spikes blood sugar levels just as sugar does, but it's harder to spoon in and doesn't dissolve as well in cold liquids. So, you tend to consume it more intentionally and consume less of it. Honey is a whole food product, and some honeys, like Ikarian heather honey, contain anti-inflammatory, anticancer, and antimicrobial properties.

Avoid sugar-sweetened sodas, teas, and fruit drinks altogether. Sugar-sweetened soda is the single biggest source of added sugars in our diet—in fact, soft drink consumption may account for 50 percent of America's weight gain since 1970. One can of soda pop alone contains around ten teaspoons of sugar. If you must drink sodas, choose diet soda or, better yet, seltzer or sparkling water.

Consume sweets as celebratory food. People in Blue Zones love sweets, but sweets (cookies, cakes, pies, desserts of many varieties) are almost always served as a celebratory food—after a Sunday meal, as part of a religious holiday, or during the village festivals. In fact, there are often special sweets for these special occasions. Limit desserts or treats to 100 calories. Eat just one serving a day or less.

Consider fruit your sweet treat in an at-home Blue Zones diet. Eat fresh fruit rather than dried fruit. Fresh fruit has more water and makes you feel fuller with fewer calories. In dried fruit, such as raisins and dates, the sugars are concentrated way beyond what you would get in a typical portion of the fruit when fresh.

Watch out for processed foods with added sugar, particularly sauces, salad dressings, and ketchup. Many contain several teaspoons of added sugar.

Watch for low-fat products, many of which are sugar-sweetened to make up for the lack of fat. Some low-fat yogurts, for instance, often contain more sugar—ounce for ounce—than soda pop.

If your sweet tooth just won't quit, try stevia to sweeten your tea or coffee. It's not an authentic part of the Blue Zones diet, of course, but it's highly concentrated, so it's probably better than refined sugar.

Snack On Nuts

Eat two handfuls of nuts per day.

A handful of nuts equals about two ounces, which appears to be the average amount that Blue Zones centenarians are eating. Here's how nuts are consumed in the various Blue Zones diets: Almonds in Ikaria and Sardinia, pistachios in Nicoya, and all nuts with the Adventists—all nuts are good. Nut-eaters on average outlive non-nut-eaters by two to three years, according to the Adventist Health Study 2.

Similarly, a recent Harvard study that followed 100,000 people for 30 years found that nut-eaters have a 20 percent lower mortality rate than non–nut-eaters. Other studies show that diets with nuts reduce "bad" LDL cholesterol by 9 percent to 20 percent , regardless of the amount of nuts consumed or the fat level in them. Other healthful ingredients in nuts include copper, fiber, folate, vitamin E, and arginine, an amino acid.

You can do it in a variety of ways.

Keep nuts around your workplace for mid-morning or mid-afternoon snacks. Take small packages for travel and car trips.

Try adding nuts or other seeds to salads and soups.

Stock up on a variety of nuts to include in your Blue Zones diet. The optimal mix: almonds (high in vitamin E and magnesium), peanuts (high in protein and folate, a B vitamin), Brazil nuts (high in selenium, a mineral thought to possibly protect against prostate cancer), cashews (high in magnesium), and walnuts (high in alpha-linoleic acid, the only omega-3 fat found in a plant- based food) (high in alpha-linoleic acid, the only omega-3 fat found in a plant- based food).

All of these nuts will help lower your cholesterol.

Incorporate nuts into regular meals as a protein source.

Eat some nuts before a meal to reduce the overall glycemic load.

Chapter Eighteen

Bread with a tangy flavor

Replace common bread with sourdough or 100 percent whole wheat bread.

Bread has been a staple in the human diet for at least 10,000 years. In three of the five Blue Zones diets, it is still a staple. While not typically used for sandwiches, it does make an appearance at most meals. But what people in Blue Zones are eating is a different food altogether from the bread that most North Americans buy. Most commercially available breads start with bleached white flour, which metabolizes q uickly into sugar. White bread delivers relatively empty calories and spikes insulin levels. In fact, white bread (together with glucose) represents the standard glycemic index score of 100, against which all other foods are measured. Refined flour is not the only problem inherent to our customary white or wheat breads. Gluten, a protein, gives bread its loft and texture, but it also creates digestive problems for some people. Bread in the Blue Zones diet is different: either whole grain or sourdough, each with its own healthful characteristics. Breads in Ikaria and Sardinia, for example, are made from a variety of 100 percent whole grains, including wheat, rye, and barley—each of which offer a wide spectrum of nutrients, such as tryptophan, an amino acid, and the minerals selenium and magnesium. Whole grains all have higher levels of fiber than most commonly used wheat flours. Interestingly, too, barley was the food most highly correlated with longevity in Sardinia. Other traditional Blue Zones breads are made with naturally occurring bacteria called lactobacilli, which "digest" the starches and glutens while making the bread rise. The process also creates an acid—the "sour" in sourdough. The result is bread with less gluten than breads labeled "gluten-free" (and about one- thousandth the amount of gluten in normal breads), with a longer shelf life and a pleasantly sour taste that most people like. Most important, traditional sourdough breads consumed in Blue Zones diets actually lower the glycemic load of meals. That means they make your entire meal healthier, slower burning, easier on your pancreas, and more likely to make calories available as energy than stored as fat. Be aware that commercial sourdough bread found in the grocery store can be very different from traditional, real sourdough, and thus may not have the same nutritional characteristics. If you want to buy true sourdough bread, shop from a reputable— probably local—bakery and ask them about their starter. A bakery that cannot answer that question is probably not making true sourdough bread, and this should not be part of your Blue Zones diet.

How you can do it:\sIf you're going to eat bread, be sure it's authentic sourdough bread like the ones they make in Ikaria. Sometimes called pain au levain, this slow-rising bread is made with lactobacteria as a rising agent, not commercial yeast.

Try to make sourdough bread yourself, and make it from an authentic sourdough starter. Ed Wood, a fellow National Geographic writer, offers some of the best information on sourdough and starters at sourdo.com.

Try a sprouted grain bread as part of your Blue Zones diet. When grains are sprouted, experts say, starches and proteins become easier to digest. Sprouted breads also offer more essential amino acids, minerals, and B vitamins than standard whole-grain varieties, and higher amounts of usable iron. Ounce for ounce, sprouts are thought to be among the most nutritious of foods.

Choose whole-grain rye or pumpernickel bread over whole wheat: They have a lower glycemic index. But look at the label. Avoid rye breads that list wheat flour as their first ingredient and look for the bread that lists rye flour as the first ingredient. Most supermarket breads aren't true rye breads.

Choose or make breads that incorporate seeds, nuts, dried fruits, and whole grains. A whole food (see the next Blue Zones food and diet rule), like flaxseeds, adds flavor, complexity, texture, and nutritional value.

Look for (or bake) coarse barley bread, with an average of 75 percent to 80 percent whole barley kernels.

In general, if you can squeeze a slice of bread into a ball, it's the kind you should avoid. Look for heavy, dense, 100 percent whole-grain breads that are minimally processed.

Go Wholly Whole

Eat foods that are recognizable for what they are.

Another definition of a "whole food" would be one that is made of a single ingredient, raw, cooked, ground, or fermented, and not highly processed. (Tofu is minimally processed, for example, while cheese doodles and frozen sausage dogs are highly processed.) Throughout the world's Blue Zones and their diets, people traditionally eat the whole food. They don't throw the yolk away to make an egg-white omelet, or spin the fat out of their yogurt, or juice the fiber-rich pulp out of their fruits. They also don't enrich or add extra ingredients to change the nutritional profile of their foods. Instead of vitamins or other supplements, they get everything they need from nutrient-dense, fiber-rich whole foods. And when they prepare dishes, those dishes typically contain a half dozen or so ingredients, simply blended together. Almost all of the food consumed by centenarians in the Blue Zones diet—up to 90 percent —also grows within a ten-mile radius of their home. Food preparation is simple. They eat raw fruits and vegetables; they grind whole grains themselves and then cook them slowly. They use fermentation—an ancient way to make nutrients bio-available—in the tofu, sourdough bread, wine, and pickled vegetables they eat. Eating only whole foods, people living in the Blue Zones rarely ingest any artificial preservatives. The foods they eat, especially the grains, are digested slowly, so blood sugar doesn't spike. Nutritional scientists are only just beginning to understand how all the elements from the entire plant (rather than isolated nutrients) work together synergistically to bring forth ultimate health. There are likely many thousands of phytonutrients—naturally occurring nutritional components of plants—yet to be discovered.

You can do it in a variety of ways.

Shop for foods at your local farmers markets or community-supported farms. Avoid factory-made foods.

Avoid foods wrapped in plastic.

Avoid food products made with more than five ingredients. Avoid pre-made or ready-to-eat meals.

Try to eat at least three Super Blue Foods daily (listed below). You don't have to eat copious amounts of these foods. But you will likely discover that these foods go far to boost your energy

and sense of vitality, so you'll be less likely to turn to the sugary, fatty, and processed stuff that gives you the immediate (and fast-fleeting) "fix."

Eat Super Blue Foods

Integrate at least three of these items into your daily Blue Zones diet to be sure you are eating plenty of whole food.

Beans—all kinds: black beans, pinto beans, garbanzo beans, black-eyed peas, lentils

Greens—spinach, kale, chards, beet tops, fennel topsTry substituting scrambled tofu for eggs as part of your Blue Zones diet.

In baking, use a q uarter cup of applesauce, a q uarter cup of mashed potatoes, or a small banana to substitute for one egg. There are also ways to use flaxseeds or agar (extracted from algae) in recipes that call for eggs.

Chapter Nineteen

Daily Dose of Beans

Eat at least a half cup of cooked beans daily.

Beans are the cornerstone of every Blue Zones diet in the world: black beans in Nicoya; lentils, garbanzo, and white beans in the Mediterranean; and soybeans in Okinawa. The long-lived populations in these Blue Zones eat at least four times as many beans as we do, on average. One five-country study, financed by the World Health Organization, found that eating 20 grams of beans daily reduced a person's risk of dying in any given year by about 8 percent . The fact is, beans represent the consummate superfood in the Blue Zones diet. On average, they are made up of 21 percent protein, 77 percent complex carbohydrates (the kind that deliver a slow and steady energy, rather than the spike you get from refined carbohydrates like white flour), and only a few percent fat. They are also an excellent source of fiber. They're cheap and versatile, come in a variety of textures, and are packed with more nutrients per gram than any other food on Earth. Humans have eaten beans for at least 8,000 years; they're part of our culinary DNA. Even the Bible's book of Daniel (1:1-21) offers a two-week bean diet to make children healthier. The Blue Zones dietary average—at least a half cup per day—provides most of the vitamins and minerals you need. And because beans are so hearty and satisfying, they'll likely push less healthy foods out of your diet. Moreover, the high fiber content in beans helps healthy probiotics flourish in the gut.

How you can do it:\sFind ways to cook beans that taste good to you and your family as part of a Blue Zones diet. Centenarians in the Blue Zones know how to make beans taste good. If you don't have favorite recipes already, resolve to try three bean recipes over the next month.

Make sure your kitchen pantry has a variety of beans to prepare. Dry beans are cheapest, but canned beans are q uicker. When buying canned beans, be sure to read the label: The only ingredients should be beans, water, spices, and perhaps a small amount of salt. Avoid the brands with added fat or sugar.

Use pureed beans as a thickener to make soups creamy and protein-rich on the Blue Zones diet.

Make salads heartier by sprinkling cooked beans onto them. Serve hummus or black bean cakes alongside salads for added texture and appeal.

Keep your pantry stocked with condiments that dress up bean dishes and make them taste delicious. Mediterranean bean recipes, for example, usually include carrots, celery, and onion, seasoned with garlic, thyme, pepper, and bay leaves. This is an easy way to mix up a Blue Zones diet.

When you go out to dinner, consider Mexican restaurants, which almost always serve pinto or black beans. Enhance the beans by adding rice, onions, peppers, guacamole, and hot sauce.

Avoid white flour tortillas. Instead, opt for corn tortillas, with which beans are consumed in Costa Rica.

Slash Sugar

Consume no more than seven added teaspoons a day.

Centenarians typically eat sweets only during celebrations. Their foods have no added sugar, and they typically sweeten their tea with honey. This adds up to about seven teaspoons of sugar a day within the Blue Zones diets. The lesson to us: Enjoy cookies, candy, and bakery items only a few times a week and ideally as part of a meal. Avoid foods with added sugar. Skip any product where sugar is among the first five ingredients listed. Limit sugar added to coffee, tea, or other foods to no more than four teaspoons per day. Break the habit of snacking on sugar-heavy sweets. Let's face it: You can't avoid sugar. It occurs naturally in fruits, vegetables, and even milk. But that's not the problem. Between 1970 and 2000, the amount of added sugars in the food supply rose 25 percent . This adds up to about 22 teaspoons of added sugar that the average American consumes daily—insidious, hidden sugars mixed into sodas, yogurts, muffins, and sauces. Too much sugar in our diet has been shown to suppress the immune system, making it harder to fend off diseases. It also spikes insulin levels, which can lead to diabetes and lower fertility, make you fat, and even shorten your life. In the Blue Zones diet, people consume about the same amount of naturally occurring sugars as North Americans do, but only about a fifth as much added sugar. The key: People in the Blue Zones consume sugar intentionally, not by habit or accident.

How you can do it:\sMake honey your go-to sweetener for a Blue Zones diet. Granted, honey spikes blood sugar levels just as sugar does, but it's harder to spoon in and doesn't dissolve as well in cold liquids. So, you tend to consume it more intentionally and consume less of it. Honey is a whole food product, and some honeys, like Ikarian heather honey, contain anti-inflammatory, anticancer, and antimicrobial properties.

Avoid sugar-sweetened sodas, teas, and fruit drinks altogether. Sugar-sweetened soda is the single biggest source of added sugars in our diet—in fact, soft drink consumption may account for 50 percent of America's weight gain since 1970. One can of soda pop alone contains around ten teaspoons of sugar. If you must drink sodas, choose diet soda or, better yet, seltzer or sparkling water.

Consume sweets as celebratory food. People in Blue Zones love sweets, but sweets (cookies, cakes, pies, desserts of many varieties) are almost always served as a celebratory food—after a Sunday meal, as part of a religious holiday, or during the village festivals. In fact, there are often special sweets for these special occasions. Limit desserts or treats to 100 calories. Eat just one serving a day or less.

Consider fruit your sweet treat in an at-home Blue Zones diet. Eat fresh fruit rather than dried fruit. Fresh fruit has more water and makes you feel fuller with fewer calories. In dried fruit, such as raisins and dates, the sugars are concentrated way beyond what you would get in a typical portion of the fruit when fresh.

Watch out for processed foods with added sugar, particularly sauces, salad dressings, and ketchup. Many contain several teaspoons of added sugar.

Watch for low-fat products, many of which are sugar-sweetened to make up for the lack of fat. Some low-fat yogurts, for instance, often contain more sugar—ounce for ounce—than soda pop.

If your sweet tooth just won't quit, try stevia to sweeten your tea or coffee. It's not an authentic part of the Blue Zones diet, of course, but it's highly concentrated, so it's probably better than refined sugar.

Snack On Nuts

Eat two handfuls of nuts per day.

A handful of nuts equals about two ounces, which appears to be the average amount that Blue Zones centenarians are eating. Here's how nuts are consumed in the various Blue Zones diets: Almonds in Ikaria and Sardinia, pistachios in Nicoya, and all nuts with the Adventists—all nuts are good. Nut-eaters on average outlive non-nut-eaters by two to three years, according to the Adventist Health Study 2.

Similarly, a recent Harvard study that followed 100,000 people for 30 years found that nut-eaters have a 20 percent lower mortality rate than non–nut-eaters. Other studies show that diets with nuts reduce "bad" LDL cholesterol by 9 percent to 20 percent , regardless of the amount of nuts consumed or the fat level in them. Other healthful ingredients in nuts include copper, fiber, folate, vitamin E, and arginine, an amino acid.

You can do it in a variety of ways.

Keep nuts around your workplace for mid-morning or mid-afternoon snacks. Take small packages for travel and car trips.

Try adding nuts or other seeds to salads and soups.

Stock up on a variety of nuts to include in your Blue Zones diet. The optimal mix: almonds (high in vitamin E and magnesium), peanuts (high in protein and folate, a B vitamin), Brazil nuts (high in selenium, a mineral thought to possibly protect against prostate cancer), cashews (high in magnesium), and walnuts (high in alpha-linoleic acid, the only omega-3 fat found in a plant- based food) (high in alpha-linoleic acid, the only omega-3 fat found in a plant- based food).

All of these nuts will help lower your cholesterol.

Incorporate nuts into regular meals as a protein source.

Eat some nuts before a meal to reduce the overall glycemic load.

Chapter Twenty

Bread with a tangy flavor

Replace common bread with sourdough or 100 percent whole wheat bread.

Bread has been a staple in the human diet for at least 10,000 years. In three of the five Blue Zones diets, it is still a staple. While not typically used for sandwiches, it does make an appearance at most meals. But what people in Blue Zones are eating is a different food altogether from the bread that most North Americans buy. Most commercially available breads start with bleached white flour, which metabolizes q uickly into sugar. White bread delivers relatively empty calories and spikes insulin levels. In fact, white bread (together with glucose) represents the standard glycemic index score of 100, against which all other foods are measured. Refined flour is not the only problem inherent to our customary white or wheat breads. Gluten, a protein, gives bread its loft and texture, but it also creates digestive problems for some people. Bread in the Blue Zones diet is different: either whole grain or sourdough, each with its own healthful characteristics. Breads in Ikaria and Sardinia, for example, are made from a variety of 100 percent whole grains, including wheat, rye, and barley—each of which offer a wide spectrum of nutrients, such as tryptophan, an amino acid, and the minerals selenium and magnesium. Whole grains all have higher levels of fiber than most commonly used wheat flours. Interestingly, too, barley was the food most highly correlated with longevity in Sardinia. Other traditional Blue Zones breads are made with naturally occurring bacteria called lactobacilli, which "digest" the starches and glutens while making the bread rise. The process also creates an acid—the "sour" in sourdough. The result is bread with less gluten than breads labeled "gluten-free" (and about one- thousandth the amount of gluten in normal breads), with a longer shelf life and a pleasantly sour taste that most people like. Most important, traditional sourdough breads consumed in Blue Zones diets actually lower the glycemic load of meals. That means they make your entire meal healthier, slower burning, easier on your pancreas, and more likely to make calories available as energy than stored as fat. Be aware that commercial sourdough bread found in the grocery store can be very different from traditional, real sourdough, and thus may not have the same nutritional characteristics. If you want to buy true sourdough bread, shop from a reputable— probably local—bakery and ask them about their starter. A bakery that cannot answer that question is probably not making true sourdough bread, and this should not be part of your Blue Zones diet.

How you can do it:\sIf you're going to eat bread, be sure it's authentic sourdough bread like the ones they make in Ikaria. Sometimes called pain au levain, this slow-rising bread is made with lactobacteria as a rising agent, not commercial yeast.

Try to make sourdough bread yourself, and make it from an authentic sourdough starter. Ed Wood, a fellow National Geographic writer, offers some of the best information on sourdough and starters at sourdo.com.

Try a sprouted grain bread as part of your Blue Zones diet. When grains are sprouted, experts say, starches and proteins become easier to digest. Sprouted breads also offer more essential amino acids, minerals, and B vitamins than standard whole-grain varieties, and higher amounts of usable iron. Ounce for ounce, sprouts are thought to be among the most nutritious of foods.

Choose whole-grain rye or pumpernickel bread over whole wheat: They have a lower glycemic index. But look at the label. Avoid rye breads that list wheat flour as their first ingredient and look for the bread that lists rye flour as the first ingredient. Most supermarket breads aren't true rye breads.

Choose or make breads that incorporate seeds, nuts, dried fruits, and whole grains. A whole food (see the next Blue Zones food and diet rule), like flaxseeds, adds flavor, complexity, texture, and nutritional value.

Look for (or bake) coarse barley bread, with an average of 75 percent to 80 percent whole barley kernels.

In general, if you can squeeze a slice of bread into a ball, it's the kind you should avoid. Look for heavy, dense, 100 percent whole-grain breads that are minimally processed.

Go Wholly Whole

Eat foods that are recognizable for what they are.

Another definition of a "whole food" would be one that is made of a single ingredient, raw, cooked, ground, or fermented, and not highly processed. (Tofu is minimally processed, for example, while cheese doodles and frozen sausage dogs are highly processed.) Throughout the world's Blue Zones and their diets, people traditionally eat the whole food. They don't throw the yolk away to make an egg-white omelet, or spin the fat out of their yogurt, or juice the fiber-rich pulp out of their fruits. They also don't enrich or add extra ingredients to change the nutritional profile of their foods. Instead of vitamins or other supplements, they get everything they need from nutrient-dense, fiber-rich whole foods. And when they prepare dishes, those dishes typically contain a half dozen or so ingredients, simply blended together. Almost all of the food consumed by centenarians in the Blue Zones diet—up to 90 percent —also grows within a ten-mile radius of their home. Food preparation is simple. They eat raw fruits and vegetables; they grind whole grains themselves and then cook them slowly. They use fermentation—an ancient way to make nutrients bio-available—in the tofu, sourdough bread, wine, and pickled vegetables they eat. Eating only whole foods, people living in the Blue Zones rarely ingest any artificial preservatives. The foods they eat, especially the grains, are digested slowly, so blood sugar doesn't spike. Nutritional scientists are only just beginning to understand how all the elements from the entire plant (rather than isolated nutrients) work together synergistically to bring forth ultimate health. There are likely many thousands of phytonutrients—naturally occurring nutritional components of plants—yet to be discovered.

You can do it in a variety of ways.

Shop for foods at your local farmers markets or community-supported farms. Avoid factory-made foods.

Avoid foods wrapped in plastic.

Avoid food products made with more than five ingredients. Avoid pre-made or ready-to-eat meals.

Try to eat at least three Super Blue Foods daily (listed below). You don't have to eat copious amounts of these foods. But you will likely discover that these foods go far to boost your energy

and sense of vitality, so you'll be less likely to turn to the sugary, fatty, and processed stuff that gives you the immediate (and fast-fleeting) "fix."

Eat Super Blue Foods

Integrate at least three of these items into your daily Blue Zones diet to be sure you are eating plenty of whole food.

Beans—all kinds: black beans, pinto beans, garbanzo beans, black-eyed peas, lentils

Greens—spinach, kale, chards, beet tops, fennel tops

Not to be confused with yams, sweet potatoes are a type of potato.

Almonds, peanuts, walnuts, sunflower seeds, Brazil nuts, and cashews are among the many types of nuts available.

The best olive oil is usually green, extra-virgin. (Because olive oil decomposes quickly, only buy a month's worth at a time.)

The best oats are slow-cooked or Irish steel-cut.

Whether in soups, as a hot cereal, or ground into bread, barley is a versatile ingredient.

All kinds of fruits

Teas made from plants or herbs

Turmeric is a spice that can be used in cooking or as a tea.

Beverage Laws in the Blue Zones

Coffee in the morning, tea in the afternoon, wine at 5 p.m., and water throughout the day. Never, ever, ever, ever, ever, ever, ever, ever, ever, ever, ever, ever,

Water, coffee, tea, and wine were the only beverages consumed in the Blue Zones. Period. (Most Blue Zone centenarians were unaware of soda pop, which accounts for roughly half of America's sugar intake.) Each option has a compelling argument.

Seven glasses of water per day are recommended by Adventists. They cite research showing that staying hydrated improves blood flow and reduces the risk of a blood clot. There is an additional benefit, in my opinion: when people drink water, they are not drinking a sugar-laden beverage (soda, energy drinks, and fruit juices) or an artificially sweetened drink, many of which are potentially carcinogenic.

Coffee is consumed in copious quantities by Sardinians, Ikarians, and Nicoyans. Coffee consumption has been linked to a reduced risk of dementia and Parkinson's disease, according to research. Furthermore, coffee in the world's Blue Zones is typically shade grown, which benefits birds and the environment—another example of how Blue Zones diet practices reflect a concern for the big picture.

Tea is consumed by residents of all Blue Zones. Green tea has been shown to reduce the risk of heart disease and several cancers, and Okinawans drink it all day long. Ikarians consume anti-inflammatory brews made from rosemary, wild sage, and dandelion.

People who drink red wine in moderation live longer than those who do not. (This isn't to say that if you don't drink now, you should start.) Most Blue Zone residents consume one to three glasses of red wine per day, usually with a meal and with friends. Wine has been shown to aid the body's absorption of plant-based antioxidants, making it an excellent addition to the Blue Zones diet. These advantages could be attributed to resveratrol, a red wine antioxidant. However, it's possible that a glass of wine at the end of the day helps to relieve stress, which is beneficial to overall health. In any case, women and men who drink more than two to three glasses per day have negative health effects. With less than one drink per day, women are more likely to develop breast cancer.

Keep a full water bottle by your bedside and at your desk or place of work.

Start your day with a cup of coffee if you want to. Coffee is lightly sweetened and served black, with no cream, in the Blue Zones diets.

Caffeine can make it difficult to sleep after mid-afternoon, so avoid it.

Green tea has about 25% the caffeine of coffee and provides a steady stream of antioxidants, so you can drink it all day.

Herbal teas like rosemary, oregano, and sage are all good choices.

Teas can be lightly sweetened with honey and stored in the fridge in a pitcher for easy access in hot weather.

Bring no soft drinks into your home.

Foods from the Blue Zones: Developing a Taste

If I've done my job correctly, I've piqued your interest with suggestions for how you can align your eating habits with those found in the Blue Zones. I've included a list of foods consumed by the world's longest-living people, as well as some tips on how to choose, prepare, and consume them. But, even though those foods make up the majority of the Blue Zones diet, what if you and your family don't like them? I could go on and on about the health benefits of broccoli and beans. If you despise broccoli and beans, however, you may eat them for a short time before becoming bored and returning to your old habits. Almost everyone is born with a sweet tooth and a dislike for bitter flavors. This is because sweetness generally denotes calories, whereas bitterness denotes toxins in some cases. Those who ate honey and berries were more likely to survive than those who ate bitter-tasting plants, including greens, which provide vitamins, minerals, and fiber and are a staple of the Blue Zones diet today. As a result, candy bars will always win out over broccoli and Brussels sprouts. Our mother's food preferences are also passed down to us at birth. We're more likely to be born with a taste for junk food if our mothers consumed salty foods high in saturated and trans fats while pregnant with us. If a woman eats a lot of garlic before giving birth, the amniotic fluid will smell like garlic, and the baby will most likely like garlic. So, if your mother wasn't a healthy eater, as many mothers after 1950 weren't, you were likely born with a disadvantage. Finally, by the age of five, most of our preferences are set. In fact, the first year of life is when children are most likely to develop new tastes. Unfortunately, most new mothers are unaware of this and feed their babies porridge or sweetened baby food, instilling in them a lifelong preference for junk food. Or they succumb to the temptation of buying salty, high-fat snacks for their children. (In the United States, 15-month-olds' favorite vegetable is French fries.) Mothers in the Blue Zones feed their babies many of the same whole foods that they eat themselves, such as rice, whole-grain porridge, and mashed-up fruits. So, how can you encourage yourself and your family to follow the Blue Zones diet? To find out, I contacted Leann L. Birch of Penn State's Department of Nutritional Sciences and Marcia Pelchat of Philadelphia's Monell Chemical Senses Center, both of whom are experts on ac q uiring tastes. Not only do we learn to like new foods throughout our lives, but there is also a science-based strategy for learning to like healthy foods.

They taught me the fundamentals of persuading children to try new, healthy foods like vegetables. These techniques can also be used by adults with minor changes.

For children, here's how to go about it:

New vegetables should have a texture that is familiar and appealing to your child because children are naturally wary of new foods. Start with new vegetables that are soft or will become soft when cooked if he or she is used to pureed foods. Present new vegetables raw if your child enjoys crispy, crunchy foods.

Introduce new foods to children when they are hungry, either before or after a meal. Don't make kids eat things they don't want to eat. You have the ability to turn them off at any time for the rest of your life.

Introduce a wide range of Blue Zones-inspired foods. Peas and carrots may be natural favorites, but broccoli and green beans may be a turnoff. Serve a half-dozen vegetables at a time in small portions, like a Blue Zones succotash, and see which ones your kids prefer. After you've figured that out, you can experiment with different ways to prepare your new favorites.

Adults can do it by figuring out what interests them. Take a cue from the above notes on how children acquire tastes and try some new vegetables when you're hungry—for example, as an appetizer before dinner.

Learn to cook in a different way. You won't eat vegetables unless you know how to make them tasty.

Attend a cooking class for vegetarians.

Organize a Blue Zones potluck dinner. With a group of your friends, go over the Blue Zones diet and food rules, as well as the list of ten Super Blue Foods. Request that everyone bring a dish that incorporates one or more of those ingredients. You can all use your culinary skills to try new plant-based foods while also strengthening your social network, which is a key goal for those looking to move their lives in the direction of the Blue Zones.

Always use four, and never use four.

The ten Blue Zones food and diet rules outlined above took a long time for my team to develop. And for some, they may be too much of a departure from the foods they have consumed their entire lives. I know what you're going through because I've been there. I used to eat whatever was available when we first started working with the city of Albert Lea. If my kitchen was stocked with ice cream and cookies, that was what I ate. I was a stalwart follower of the "See Food Diet": See food, eat it. I knew we needed to start with some simple guidelines. I brought together some of the smartest people I could find, and we started by figuring out how to make kitchens healthier. We reasoned that if we could identify the four best foods from the Blue Zones diet to always have on hand, and the four worst foods to never have on hand—and create a nudge—we might be able to get people to eat better. I included myself among the potential benefactors.

Cornell's Brian Wansink, the University of Minnesota's Leslie Lytle, and a few others got together to brainstorm the foods that were best and worst for us. We established a few criteria:

The "Always" foods had to be readily available and affordable.

The "Always" foods had to taste good and be versatile enough to include in most meals.

The "To Avoid" foods had to be highly correlated with obesity, heart disease, or cancer as well

as a constant temptation in the average American diet.

Strong evidence had to back up all food designations as "Always" and "To Avoid".

Chapter Twenty-one

Four Always

Remembering four food groups might be an easier starting point than remembering all the foods prepared in the Blue Zones diet. Here's our list. 100 percent Whole Wheat Bread: We figured it could be toasted in the morning and become part of a healthy sandwich at lunch. While not, perhaps, the perfect longevity food, it could help force white breads out of the diet and be an important step toward a healthier Blue Zones diet for most Americans.

Nuts: We know that nut-eaters outlive those who don't eat nuts. Nuts come in a variety of flavors, and they're full of nutrients and healthy fat that satiate your appetite. The ideal snack is a two-ounce mix of nuts (about a handful) (about a handful). Ideally, you should keep small two-ounce packages on hand. Small quantities are best, since the oils in nuts degrade (oxidize) (oxidize). Larger quantities can be stored in the refrigerator or freezer for a couple of months.

Beans: I argue that beans of every type are the world's greatest longevity foods. They're cheap, versatile, and full of antioxidants, vitamins, and fiber, and they can be made to taste delicious. It's best to buy dry beans and it's easy to cook them, but low-sodium canned beans in non-BPA cans are okay too. Learn how to cook with beans and keep them on hand, and you'll make a big leap toward living longer with a Blue Zones diet.

Your Favorite Fruit: Buy a beautiful fruit bowl, place it in the middle of your kitchen (either the counter, center island, or table—wherever gets the most traffic), and place it under a light. Research shows that we really do eat what we see, so if chips are always in plain sight, that's what we'll eat. But if there is a fruit you like and keep in plain sight all the time, you'll eat more of it and be healthier for it. Don't bother buying a fruit you think you ought to eat but really don't like.

Four to Avoid

By the same token, remembering four rules about which foods to avoid to help you Blue Zone your refrigerator and kitchen cupboard might make the process easier. We're not saying that you can never treat yourself to these foods. In fact, if you love any of these foods and they make you happier, you should absolutely indulge occasionally. But save them for celebrations or, at the very least, make sure you have to go out to get them. Just don't bring them into your home, and you'll cut many of these toxic foods that don't exist in the Blue Zones diet out of your diet without too much grief.

Sugar-Sweetened Beverages:\sHarvard's Willett has estimated that 50 percent of America's caloric gain is directly attributable to the empty calories and li q uefied sugar that come in sodas and boxed juices. Would you ever put ten teaspoons of sugar on your cereal? Probably not. But that's how much sugar you consume on average when you drink a 12-ounce can of soda pop.

Salty Snacks: We spend about $6 billion a year on potato chips—the food (not coincidentally, perhaps) most highly correlated with obesity (though fried pork rinds are closing in fast) (though fried pork rinds are closing in fast). Almost all chips and crackers deliver high doses of salt, preservatives, and highly processed grains that\sq uickly metabolize to sugar. They've also been carefully formulated to be optimally crunchy and tasty and to deliver a sultry mouth feel. In other words, they're engineered to be irresistible. So how do you resist them? Don't have them in your home!

Processed Meats: A recent gold-standard epidemiology study followed more than half a million people for decades and found that those who consumed high amounts of sausages, salami, bacon, lunch meats, and other highly processed meats had the highest rates of cancers and heart disease. Again, the threat is twofold here. The nitrates and other preservatives used in these meat products are known carcinogens. They do the job, though, and preserve the products well, which means that processed meats are readily available on the shelf at home or in the store, right there for snacking or a q uick meal—something that doesn't happen in Blue Zones households and diets.

Packaged Sweets: Like salty snacks, cookies, candy bars, muffins, granola bars, and even energy bars all deliver a punch of insulin-spiking sugars. We're all genetically hardwired to crave sweets, so we instinctively want to satiate a craving by ripping open a package of cookies and digging in. Lessons from the Blues Zones diet would tell us that if you want to bake some cookies or a cake and have it around, okay. If you want to enjoy the occasional baked treat at your corner bakery, fine. But don't stock your pantry with any wrapped sugary snacks. For your convenience, I've brought together all the longevity foods into a single list, below. Pick as many

as you can, learn to prepare them, stick with them for the long run, and see how good they make you feel.

Longevity Superfoods from the World's Blue Zones Diets

Vegetables\sFennel\sKombu (seaweed) (seaweed) Wakame (seaweed) (seaweed)

Potatoes

Shiitake mushrooms S q uash

Sweet potatoes Wild greens Yams

Fruits Avocados Bananas Bitter melons Lemons Papayas

Pejivalles (peach palms) (peach palms) Plantains\sTomatoes

Black beans are a kind of legume.

Black-eyed peas are a kind of pea that grows in the southern United States Fava beans are a kind of chickpea.

Beans that are already cooked

Chapter Twenty-two

Nuts besides almonds

Whole-grain bread with barley Oatmeal maize nixtamal brown rice brown rice maize maize maize maize maize maize maize maize maize

Nuts and seeds are two types of nuts and seeds that may be found in nature.

Salmon with Less Fat Tofu prepared with soy milk

Feta cheese made from dairy products Cheese Pecorino

Oils added

Olive oil is a kind of vegetable oil that comes

Beverages Coffee Green tea is a beverage made from the leaves of Wine (red) Water

Seasonings and sweeteners are two types of ingredients that may be used to make food taste better

Mediterranean herbs Garlic Honey Turmeric, milk thistle

What gives these individuals in the Blue Zones the ability to live such long lives?

There's no doubting that genetics have a role in deciding how long you live, but research suggests that genetics only account for roughly 20% to 30% of lifespan. 70 to 80 percent of your longevity is controlled by nutrition, community, lifestyle, and other environmental variables. While many people believe that what they eat has the greatest impact on weight gain and illness risk, Jaime Schehr, N.D., R.D., a New York-based nutritionist, argues that lifestyle factors and nutrition are inextricably linked when it comes to longevity.

Buettner discovers nine characteristics across Blue Zones, dubbed the "Power 9," that directly contribute to the reduction of obesity and metabolic disorders, as well as an increase in life expectancy, according to research. These are the secrets to a healthy, longer life.

Make your own movements.

The world's longest-lived individuals are surrounded by circumstances that promote and require them to move without thinking about it: more walking and carrying items, less weight lifting and marathon running. Any activity is beneficial, but basic physical work such as mowing the lawn, gardening, and making things is preferable.

Get a sense of direction.

It's known as "Ikigai" in Okinawa and "plan de vida" in Nicoya; both terms mean "why I get up in the morning." "Those who lived the longest have a strong sense of purpose," Buettner adds.

Don't worry about it.

Even those who live in the Blue Zones are subject to stress. However, unlike the majority of us, these centenarians have components of their daily routine that help them relax. Adventists pray, Ikarians slumber, and Sardinians sip wine. And they all have a support system (more on that in a moment), explains the author.

The Functional Medical Institute in Tulsa, OK, was founded by Mark Sherwood, N.D.

Reduce your intake.

The Okinawans have an old adage that says they should stop eating when their tummies are 80 percent full. Sherwood points out that people in the Blue Zones eat their smallest—and last—meal in the late afternoon or early evening, a pattern that is repeated in intermittent fasting.

Plants for meat trade.

Beans, unprocessed grains such as oats and barley, greens, potatoes, nuts and seeds, fruits, and herbs are all common foods in the Blue Zones. It's hardly surprise that the world's oldest individuals follow a plant-based diet, which has been shown to reduce your risk of practically every illness. They do ingest animal protein, but only in modest amounts, according to Schehr. People in the Blue Zones consume meat just five times a month, mostly pork. (As for the iron levels, what's up with that?) The mineral is abundant in certain meat-free diets.) "Disorders such as diabetes, obesity, heart disease, cancer, and inflammatory diseases have all been related to the use of empty calories, excess calories, large levels of sugar, and animal proteins," adds Schehr.

Chapter Twenty-three

It's time to celebrate.

People drink moderately and frequently in every Blue Zone except Loma Linda, California. While it is well known that moderate drinkers outlast nondrinkers, it is critical to stress the word "moderate"—one drink per day for women. That cup is usually filled with red wine and consumed with companions or food in these countries (just be sure to steer clear of these vino mistakes).

Belong.

Except for five of the 263 centenarians interviewed for Buettner's book, every one of the 263 centenarians belonged to a faith-based group. It doesn't matter what denomination you belong to, but studies indicate that attending faith-based services four times a month may add four to fourteen years to your life expectancy.

Always prioritize your family.

Successful centenarians keep their elderly parents and grandparents close by or at home, which reduces health concerns such as depression in the offspring. They also commit to a life partner, which studies suggest may extend one's lifespan, and spend time and affection in their children, which motivates the children to care for their older parents when the time comes.

Locate a group.

According to a 2015 meta-analysis from Brigham Young University, loneliness has just as much (if not more) of an impact on health and mortality risk as the top killers in America: smoking, obesity, alcohol addiction, and exercise. According to the same research, those with strong social ties are 50% less likely to die over time than those with less social ties. This is something that residents of the Blue Zones are well aware of: Moais, for example, are groups of five friends who make a lifelong commitment to one another. "More chances for connections and support are available as a result of belonging to a community. It is possible to find hope through having someone to speak to, share life with, and play with. This optimism is fueled by the fact that someone has a cause to live (e.g., someone needs you), which makes stress much easier to handle "Sherwood is quoted as saying

What is the mechanism?

The anti-inflammatory advantages of Blue Zone people's food choices, according to research, are a powerful reason underlying increased lifespan and reduced chronic disease risk. While these centenarians' diets aren't entirely plant-based, they certainly eat a lot of them. Blue Zone residents place a high value on vegetables, particularly those produced at home, since they contain a wealth of vitamins, minerals, fiber, and antioxidants. In these communities, beans and lentils are excellent plant-based protein sources. Legumes, like vegetables, are high in fiber, which offers a variety of health advantages, including lowering the risk of heart disease and aiding in blood sugar regulation. Olive oil, which is high in heart-healthy fatty acids and antioxidants, is utilized in various Blue Zone locations. People in the blue zone consume little red meat and only three times a week eat little servings of seafood. These people still enjoy sweets and other meals in moderation, but they eat prudently and do not overeat. Weight may be kept under control and chronic illness can be avoided by practicing moderation and balance with dietary choices, particularly by adhering to guidelines like the hara hachi bu concept, which the Okinawans practice.

Chapter Twenty-four

Pasta with Cherry Tomatoes and Basil in One Pot in the Instant Pot

INGREDIENTS

1 tbsp extra virgin olive oil (optional), plus more as needed

1 tblsp. chopped yellow onion

4 garlic cloves (slices)

14 teaspoon flakes de pimentón

Uncooked short pasta, 1 pound (450 grams) (such as penne, fusilli, or bowtie)

a pinch of salt

water, 4–5 cups

Cherry tomatoes, 1 pint (551ml)

1 bunch torn or sliced fresh basil

14 cup capers, rinsed

1 vegan Parmesan cheese cup, shredded

ground just now

Chapter Twenty-five

Salad of Sardinian oranges and fennel with citrus vinaigrette

DIRECTIONS

Select Sauté (Medium) on the Instant Pot and heat the oil in the inner pot, if used, until it is hot. (If you don't have any water in the bottom of the pot, you may dry sauté in it.) 3 to 5 minutes until the onion is cooked and brown. Sauté for another minute with the garlic and pepper. Cancel the action.

In the inner pot of the Instant Pot, place the pasta. Add the salt and water until the pasta is just covered, about 14 inch (0.5 cm) above the water level. Without stirring, place the tomatoes on top.

Make sure the steam release valve on the Instant Pot is set to the sealing position. Select Pressure Cook (Low) and, rounding down, set the cook time to half of the pasta package's cook time. Set the cook time for 5 minutes if the pasta packet says to cook it for 10 to 12 minutes on the burner.

Quickly release the pressure and gently remove the cover after the cook time is finished. Stir in the capers and fresh basil. If preferred, add a drizzle of olive oil. Serve right away with a sprinkle of Parmesan and seasonings to suit.

INGREDIENTS:

1 trimmed and finely sliced fennel bulb

2 to 3 peeled oranges

optional 2 tbsp craisins

1-2 tablespoons olive oil with lime infusion

1 tablespoon vinegar (lemon or pineapple)

2 or 3 mint sprigs for decoration to taste, pepper

DIRECTIONS

Arrange the chopped fennel slices on a serving platter to serve.

Section the oranges and set them on top of the fennel.

Craisins on top

Some fennel fronds should be saved and reserved for garnishing the salad's top. Using lime oil as a finishing touch,

vinegars made from pineapples

INGREDIENTS IN OKINAWAN MUSSEL SOUP

34 cup chopped leeks or 1 small onion

1 tsp. oil

1 tsp sodium

112 cup shiitake mushrooms (or 12 cup shiitake, enoki, and Shemeji mushrooms combined)

1 tsp. grated ginger

2 c soy milk, unsweetened

bay leaf (one)

miso paste, 1 tbsp

Chapter Twenty-six

NICOYA CHUNKY VEGAN SOUP

DIRECTIONS

5-6 minutes in a big saucepan, stir fried onion with a touch of salt until tender.

Continue to sauté mushrooms until they are tender.

Bring to a simmer with the ginger, soy milk, and bay leaf.

3 minutes on low heat

INGREDIENTS IN

1 tbsp. olive oil (extra virgin)

2 garlic cloves, chopped

1 tblsp. diced onion

2 chayote squash, peeled and diced into 12-inch cubes

2 lbs. yuca, peeled and diced into 12-inch dice*

3 small yellow squash or zucchini, peeled and diced into 12 inch chunks

3 peeled and diced potatoes (12 inch)

3 peeled and diced carrots (12 inch)

1 ayote s q uash**, peeled, seeded, and diced into 12-inch chunks

4 peeled and diced mini sweet peppers

1 sprig celery (chopped)

3–4 quarts vegetable broth

To taste, season with salt

DIRECTIONS

In a soup pot, heat the oil and stir-fry the onion and garlic for 3-4 minutes.

Cover and cook on low for 30-40 minutes, or until the vegetables are soft.

Before serving, season with a pinch of salt.

Remove the bay leaf, turn off the heat, and stir in the miso just before serving.

Chapter Twenty-seven

Conclusion

Last but not least, Your Personal Blue Zone (goals for a way of life of health and longevity you are committed to lead.) Take advantage of the nine lessons that will help you gain valuable years (canvassed in "Your Personal Blue Zone" chapter.) It's crucial that you only try three lessons at a time...start with three! You'll run out of time if you try to tackle all nine at once. Make a list of the specific lessons you'll learn and how you'll learn them.

CPSIA information can be obtained
at www.ICGtesting.com
Printed in the USA
LVHW051830300322
714790LV00007B/495